Bodybuilding

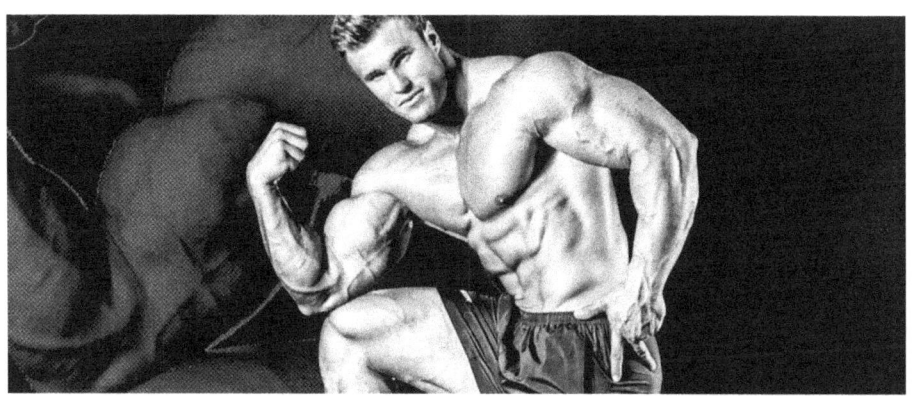

The Guide to Build the
Ultimate Body

Arnold Yates

table of contents

CHAPTER 1

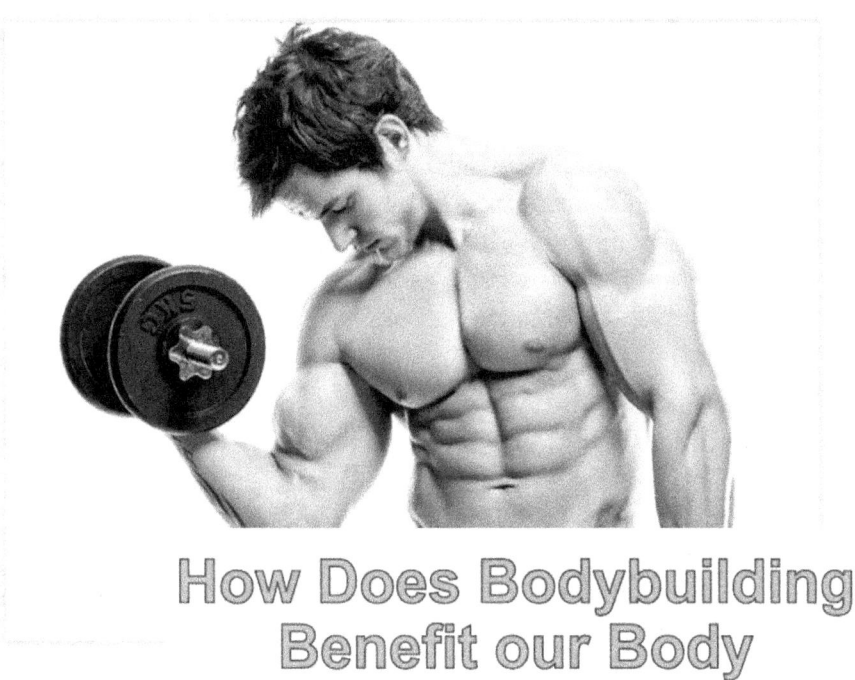

How Does Bodybuilding Benefit our Body

Building up the muscles and getting in shape is the dream of each one of us. Besides a good health sign, a body in good shape becomes ideal and attractive. In bodybuilding, we train our body to build muscles by promoting and boosting up natural muscle growth through wisely planned exercises and healthy eating.

In older times, shaping or building up the body was considered as a sport, but now it has become a craze, a trend or a fashion more than a sport or professionalism. Actually, bodybuilding is a technique to build beautiful and powerful muscles through progressive resistance exercise.

It is also said that bodybuilding not only builds great muscles but also trains minds. In bodybuilding, progression day after day gives you self-confidence and self-esteem that not only strengthens your body but also your mind. Being a fitness trainer, I myself trained by attitude while training my body.

In the beginning, you may find bodybuilding a daunting experience due to its traditional tiresome routine and your mindset towards bodybuilding. If you have a little knowledge about bodybuilding, then you will soon tired of your routine workouts and consider it a puzzle that you cannot solve.

Contrary to this, if you have great enthusiasm for bodybuilding and you have a sufficient knowledge about this sport and benefits, then the odd of success is 80% (as there is a lot more to know about bodybuilding to get 100% success in this field like Eugen Sandow, Arnold Schwarzenegger, Ronnie Coleman, jay cutler and many more). Through proper workouts and planning, you can get an inspiring and attractive body.

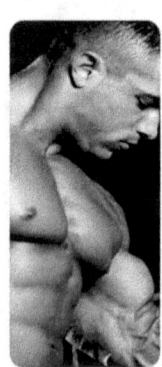

The true Understanding with Bodybuilding

If you think that bodybuilding is more than about hugely muscled body then you are on the right track with a little knowledge about bodybuilding. In fact, bodybuilding is an art in which you engrave or draw muscles through a certain duration of sincere training, intellectually or emotionally binding yourself with your passion and the right guidance.

The early concept of bodybuilding started from lifting stones in ancient Greece and Egypt. Greek people were excelled in shaping their bodies, though with no very good techniques. The people of that time used to focus on getting stronger instead of defining their muscles.

The modern bodybuilding is the developed form of ancient bodybuilding. The professional bodybuilding developed in the 19th century in Europe (England). Eugen Sandow is considered the father of the bodybuilding what it is today.

Sandow led the foundation of posing the body muscles before the audience and somewhat promoted it to the next generations. Bodybuilding got a wide fame in the 1950s and 1960s when the international federation of bodybuilding was founded.

In the 1970s, Arnold Schwarzenegger was a popular and the most famous bodybuilder of that ear. Many anabolic steroids and some other similar substances were introduced in that time and got fame in a short time.

Professionally, bodybuilding requires planning, great struggle, stamina, power, different techniques and enthusiasm. The history has seen a number of great bodybuilders who have proved themselves the remarkable and incredible persons of their age/ era. They had devoted all they had for their profession and success. They used to train their muscles with an already set battle plan for their workouts.

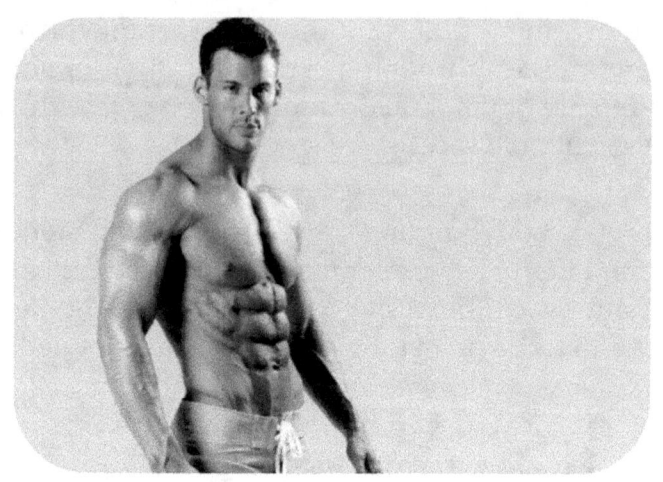

How does Bodybuilding Benefit our Muscles

Besides being a professional sport, bodybuilding benefits in various ways such as it builds bigger muscles and burn fat to give you a hot and stunning body. The weight training makes you better looking and different from others. Healthy activities like exercises are a sure way to stay fit and healthy. The benefits of exercises like weight training cannot be described in words only. You can understand the meaning of staying healthy if you have ever suffered from a health condition.

Here are some of the benefits of weight training or bodybuilding:

Improved mental and physical health
Bigger body muscles along with increased physical strength

Enhanced self-confidence and self-esteem

Stay fit and healthy for life and say good-bye to diseases such as diabetes, cardiovascular diseases, chronic stress, low energy level and hypertension

An improved production of hormones

Increased body mass due to stronger muscles and harder bones

Better posture and reduced body fat that affects your personality

Reduced risks of infectious diseases

summary

Through proper training, you learn how to make a right decision at the right time. As weight training, bodybuilding exercises or resistance training, involve precise controlled movements for each muscle group, therefore, these exercises increase the range of motion and strength of the muscles involved in exercises. Exercises performed for building up your muscles increase resting metabolic rate and help your body in burning unnecessary body fat.

A better body shape not only gives you a better pose while sitting and standing, but also boost up self-confidence or self-esteem. An improved overall health through weight training leads to produce newer and stronger muscles that are larger than before (due to the increased number of muscle tissues).

In bodybuilding, we train our muscles through harder means to boost up muscle building hormones and muscle building process. The outmoded muscles are damaged during high-intensity exercises and are naturally repaired while we rest. The outmoded/damaged muscles are utilized or removed from the body via different processes and new muscles take the place of them that are increased in number and stronger than before. That is how bodybuilding improves and strengthens our body muscles.

Weight training for building up muscles improves our overall health that leads to a life free of chronic diseases such as cardiac health problems, diabetes, obesity and many more. Exercises are the best way to fight against chronic health conditions in a natural way.

In bodybuilding, a bodybuilder trains his or her muscles to promote the production of growth hormone and other hormones that are responsible for muscle growth and strength.

Through the combination of aerobic and anaerobic exercises, a bodybuilder maintains his/her weight by burning unnecessary body fat and by developing stronger and well-defined muscles. Proper training of bodybuilding makes you bigger, stronger and unique not the giant.

CHAPTER 2

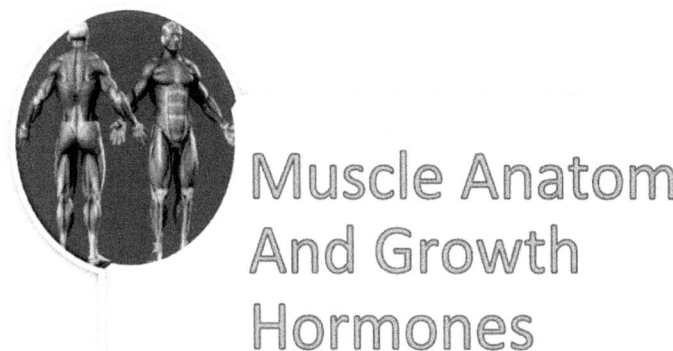

Muscle Anatomy And Growth Hormones

TYPES OF MUSCLES

Our body contains a variety of muscles that are of different shapes and characteristics. These muscles are different from each other with respect to the different tasks and structure such as cardiac muscles, smooth muscles, and skeletal muscles.

CARDIAC MUSCLES

Cardiac muscles (involuntary) are responsible for the contraction and relaxation of heart in order to generate heartbeats and are found in heart only.

SMOOTH MUSCLES

Smooth muscles are found within the walls of our body organs such as stomach, esophagus, blood vessels, urethra, uterus, intestines, bladder, and bronchi.

SKELETAL MUSCLES

Skeletal muscles are the muscles, which are responsible for skeletal movements like locomotion and are responsible for maintaining body posture. Our skeletal muscles control every action that we consciously perform such as walking, sitting, running and eating, because these are the only voluntary muscles or striated muscle that can be controlled voluntarily in our body. Skeletal muscles are attached to two moving bones across a joint in order to perform the motion of the organs containing bones closer to each other. Through a continuous resistance training, skeletal muscles are capable of adapting to a particular situation or shape after. With respect to the speed of twitch skeletal muscles are divided into two types;

- Slow twitch

- Fast twitch

Slow twitch muscles exert little force while prolonged contracting. These muscles are red in color as they rich with capillaries, mitochondria and myoglobin. Slow twitch muscles can carry excessive oxygen and thus they sustain aerobic activity and are powered by aerobic reactions using fats or carbohydrates as fuel.

Fast twitch muscles can contract quickly with more force but fatigue soon/rapidly, are responsible for muscle strength and increase in mass. Fast twitch muscles are powered by anaerobic reactions.

Understanding the Muscle Growth Hormone

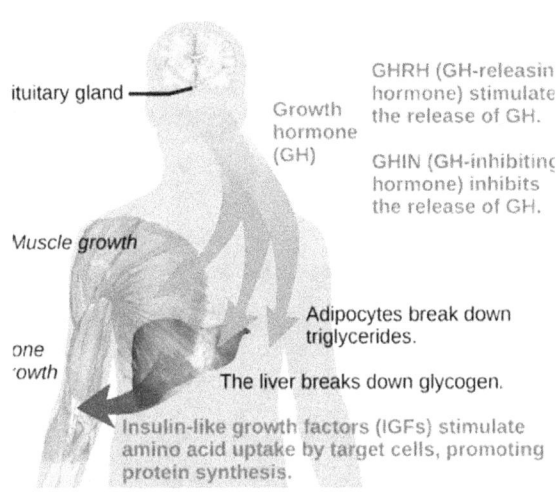

ituitary gland

Growth hormone (GH)

GHRH (GH-releasin hormone) stimulate the release of GH.

GHIN (GH-inhibitinc hormone) inhibits the release of GH.

Muscle growth

Adipocytes break down triglycerides.

one
'owth

The liver breaks down glycogen.

Insulin-like growth factors (IGFs) stimulate amino acid uptake by target cells, promoting protein synthesis.

There are different types of hormones that stimulate our different moods and body systems to function properly. Our body hormones play a key role in muscle growth. In general, hormones are the secretions of secretors called glands. The hormones responsible for growth are generally known as growth hormone or stress hormones.

Besides muscle growth, growth hormone are also responsible for bone growth and other functions as they stimulate other glands to secret their secretions. The amount of a hormone secreted by a gland depends upon the gender, physical activities (exercises and routine works) and foods we eat. Being a master gland, pituitary gland stimulates or regulates other glands functioning under the control of pituitary gland.

The master gland stimulates growth hormone by signaling them for secreting their hormones and is responsible for physical growth itself. Growth hormone increases the concentration of glucose and free fatty acids in our body, which have muscle-building effects on our body.

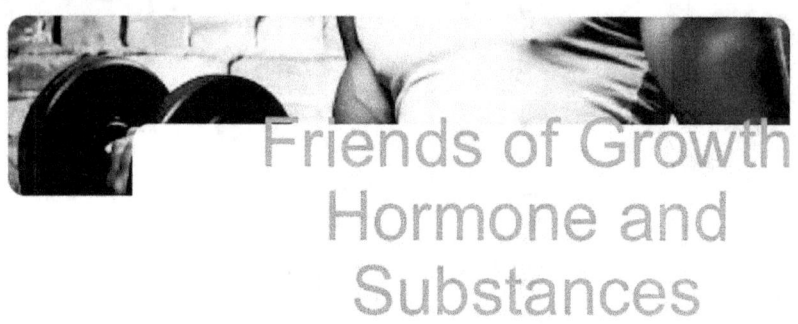

Friends of Growth Hormone and Substances

Our body have some factors that work like growth hormone. These factors are known as hepatocytes growth factors and fibroblast growth factor. Growth hormone or hormones like substances such as Hepatocyte growth factor (HGF) and Fibroblast growth factor (FGF) stimulate our satellite cells. Satellite cells of our body are the cells that are stimulated by growth factors and migrate to the point of action.

HEPATOCYTE GROWTH FACTOR

Hepatocyte growth factor regulates satellite cell activity and is responsible for causing satellite cells to migrate to damaged muscles in order to repair them and to regenerate damaged muscles.

FIBROBLAST GROWTH FACTOR

Fibroblast growth factor repairs damaged or injured muscles after practicing high-intensity exercises and getting hurt. Fibroblast growth factor has the regulatory and stimulating effect on our body's repair system that's why fibroblast growth factor is involved in angiogenesis (wound healing by forming new blood vessels) and after exercise.

TESTOSTERONE AND MUSCLE GROWTH

Testosterone is an anabolic steroid hormone and is secreted by the testicles and ovaries of male and female respectively. In males, testosterone develops male reproductive tissues (testis and prostate), increases hair growth and increase muscle and bone mass. The level of testosterone released in males is greater than the female of the same age.

Testosterone being an anabolic steroid has anabolic effects such as, responsible for linear growth, the growth of muscles, muscle strength and increased bone mass and strength. Testosterone is also involved in bone maturation. Testosterone increases protein within cells and in skeletal muscles and thus, they add additional mass to our body if stimulated by exercise and other physical activities.

SYNTHETIC GROWTH HORMONE AND ITS DOWNSIDE

There are countless people who are using synthetic growth hormones and some severely harmful steroids to get in shape and to build muscles in quicker short time to attract and impress other people. In fact, these people are killing themselves by building their muscles through unnatural means.

Our body is designed to utilize natural things either they are hormones naturally produced by our body glands or they are foods obtained from natural means like plants and animals, but in some children and diseased people with impaired hormone level for their proper growth, are prescribed to take synthetic growth hormone.

These unnaturally produced or man-made (synthetic) hormones are manufactured for the treatment purposes, not for the fancier people. These synthetic hormones if taken by a healthy person without any medical purpose or without the prescription of a health expert or physician can harm severely or leave untreatable side effects. Therefore, we need to stick to promote our body system to prepare this growth hormone naturally for muscle growth through healthy means such as exercising and healthy eating/diet.

CONCLUSION

Muscle growth rate can be increased in a healthy way through proper diet and exercise in a well-structured way. Our body hormones are the most important factors that promote muscle growth naturally because they help in building up strong and healthy muscles rapidly. We can regulate the secretion of this growth hormone by healthy eating and some effective physical activities. In males, muscle growth rate is higher than females due to the change in gender and other physical needs and abilities. If your body does not secrete sufficient amounts of growth hormone or hormones like substances, then supplementation can be adopted along with an effective and professional exercise plan. If somehow supplementation is necessary, then you should consult an authentic physician or a nutritionist before you start supplementation based on self-prescription.

CHAPTER 3

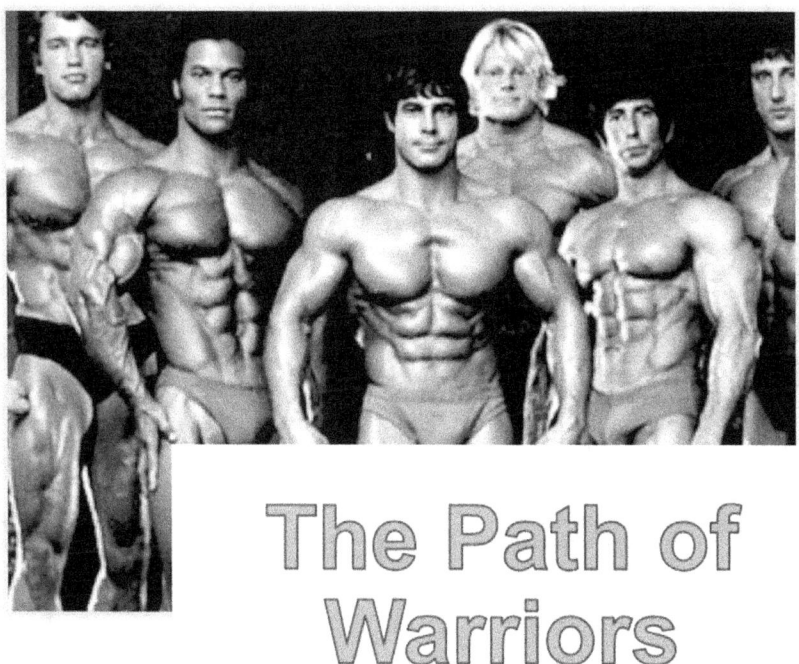

The Path of Warriors

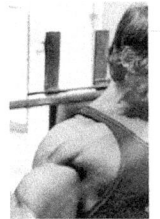

Training and Workout Strategies of Legends

The history is the spectator of the secrets workout strategies of the successful legends of bodybuilding such as Eugen Sandow, Arnold Schwarzenegger, Ronnie Coleman, jay cutler. Some of the secret workout strategies of these great legends of bodybuilding who devoted their lives for the success are given in short ideas:

GET A LEANER BODY FIRST

Burn as much calories as you can, in the beginning, to get leaner and a well-shaped body. A proper training is a key to building and preserve muscles. Almost the majority of the popular professional bodybuilders had the same training technique. According to the great legends of bodybuilding, weight training with high intensity, three times a week (non-consecutive days) works great to build bigger quality muscles and leaner body.

Do a very few isolation workouts and focus on compound movements like pull ups, lat pull downs, squats, Romanian deadlifts, bench press, dips, shoulder press, cable back rows and barbell back rows.

CARDIO

The right type of cardio will help you to get a lean body with well-defined muscles. Prioritize shorter high-intensity sessions over longer low-intensity sessions at the end of the weight lifting days or on off days to get expected results in quicker short time.

TRAIN BIGGER MUSCLES BEFORE SMALLER

ll legendary men believed that larger muscle groups should be trained before the smaller ones. Nowadays in the gyms, many young persons can be seen doing zigzag training. You can observe them training their calves before quads and biceps before back muscles. In fact, back muscles are larger than biceps that's why back muscles need to be trained before biceps. Likewise, performing lighter exercises before heavier exercises is the wrong side of exercises. According to Arnold's way of exercising and some other most popular bodybuilders, heavier movements should be performed before lighter movements in the training session such as deadlifts before lat pull downs, the squats before lunges and the bench press before the flyes.

TAKE A START WITH CORE EXERCISES

Cables, machines and isolation exercises do not require enough body balance, because in these exercises, less or no body balance is required. On the other hand, back rows, overhead press, deadlifts and squats should be performed first, as more technique and body balance is required to perform these exercises correctly.

COMPETE YOUR YESTERDAY

Always try to do your best on the next day of your training session to defeat your yesterday training. It means that you need to perform with more intensity and enthusiasm better than you did yesterday. This is the best way to improve in days instead of months and this is the secret way of training of legendary bodybuilders of the past time.

GIVE FIRST PRIORITY TO MORE TECHNICAL WORKOUTS

If you study some of the most popular and professional Olympic award-winning bodybuilders, then you will come to know that they all have some secret ways of building up monster muscles like batman, superman, and other superheroes. I have mentioned some of the most important key elements of building up bigger muscles with a leaner body. Practicing technical exercises that require more coordination, power, timing, speed and technique before simple exercises is the easy way to keep your body energetic throughout your training session.

BE CREATIVE

After learning sufficient knowledge and techniques of bodybuilding exercises, you can slightly vary the angle of your exercise for better tension and stretch in your muscles. You can increase tension in your muscles by changing your grip and foot stance.

ALTERNATE COMBINATIONS

Your bodybuilding career is going on the wheels of your exercise routine. So, keep changing these tires to run this career safely. I mean change your exercise routine by making a little bit change in your routine combination. Performing flat bench and incline bench press one combination and incline bench press and parallel bar dips another combination is a good change you can make in your exercise plan.

NEVER IGNORE YOUR WEAK POINTS

The majority of the new age bodybuilders build their program around their stronger areas and almost neglect their weak points. Prioritizing your weak points to bring them up is hard to do, but it is fruitful. All the legendary bodybuilders prioritize their weak points to fight against their weakness and to bring them up.

PLAN MUST ADDRESS CURRENT REQUIREMENTS

It is important to modify your training plan over time as you progress in order to stay motivated. You should not use the same plan that you did when you were a beginner. Your exercise plan must address your present requirements in the ever-progressing journey of bodybuilding.

SELF-DISOBEDIENCE

Try to control your inner desires to quit the training for today, keep yourself strong, and compel us to follow your routine plans strictly. Self-disobedience is key to success because the person inside you sometimes wants to do something you should not do at that moment.

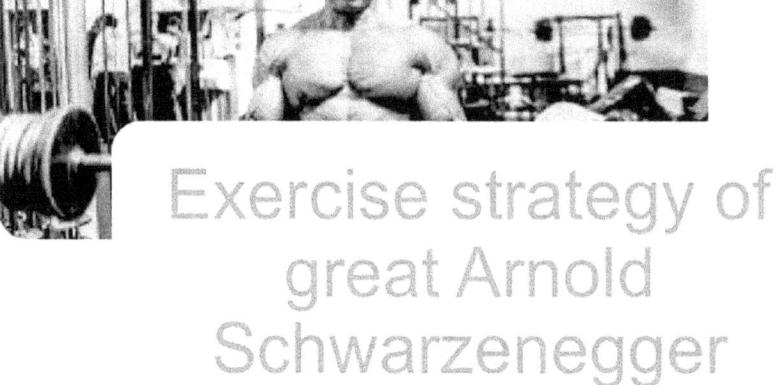

Exercise strategy of great Arnold Schwarzenegger

Arnold Schwarzenegger being a most popular and the best bodybuilder of his age believed in core free weight exercises, heavy weights, high-intensity techniques and high volume exercises.

If you want to train like Arnold and other popular legendary bodybuilders, then follow this training strategy;

- ♥ **Lifting heavy weights**: training with heavy muscles with a proper technique results in bigger and stronger muscles. In this training session, you have to lift the weight heavy enough you that you can lift hardly or your muscles unable to lift that weight for more than 8 times.

- ♥ **High Volume:** Train a target muscle group with a high number of sets - usually 20-30 sets per muscle group is the most favorite and effective exercise of all the great bodybuilders.

- ♥ **Minimize machine and isolation exercises:** Compound free weight exercises such as parallel bar dips and barbell/ dumbbell shoulder press , pull ups, deadlifts, squats, barbell and dumbbell shrugs, cable lat pull downs and cable seated rows are the best maneuver to build a super human body. Minimize machine and isolation exercises, because these exercises are not relatively effective.

- ♥ **Experimentation:** experiment with your training by slightly changing your grips, foot stance and angles to exert more force and stretch your muscles like Arnold did.

- ♥ **Adopt good habits:** selecting healthy foods rich with nutrients and avoid eating bad foods high in (calories but low in nutrition), getting enough sleep and expanding your social circle inspire you to become more popular among them that instills self-confidence and self-esteem.

- ♥ **Working in a rep range:** working in a rep range helps you in building healthier and stronger muscles in quicker short time. According to experienced and successful bodybuilders like Arnold, a tough set of 6-8 reps is as hard as doing a tough set of 20 reps with lighter weight. Doing 20 reps with much lighter weights is not sufficient to build bigger muscles that you can build with heavy weights with 6-8 reps.

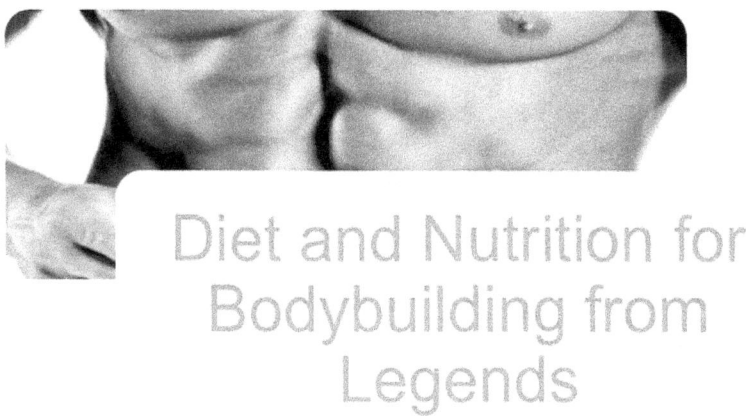

Diet and Nutrition for Bodybuilding from Legends

If you are working on developing your muscles, you most likely already know that working out, by itself, isn't sufficient. Diet plan is also crucial. Eating like a body builder can help you get ripped and lose extra weight if you merge this diet with the right workout routine. The basic idea is to eat a diet full of protein and fiber, and low in carbohydrates and fat. This diet also includes eating much more often.

When you consider the diet plans of the top body builders, you'll observe that all of them have different diet plans with different meals, different meal timings and different macros but they stick to the same fundamental principles. Let's have a look at what some of the stars did with their diet.

ARNOLD SCHWARZENEGGER

The 7-time Mr. Olympia would mainly concentrate on eating whole, natural foods and staying away from foods that were highly processed. A few of the principles he suggested are:

♥ Eat 5-6 smaller meals each day

♥ Eat carbohydrates 30 minutes after exercising

- ♥ Consume 30 to 50 grms of proteins with every meal
- ♥ Not avoid saturated fat due to the fact they boost hormonal levels
- ♥ Eat no more than 3 egg per day
- ♥ Replace beef and pork with poultry and fish
- ♥ Stay away from sugar — it has empty calories; eat vegetables and fruit for carbohydrates alternatively
- ♥ Use supplements and protein shakes to get the necessary daily amount of protein

RONNIE COLEMAN

Coleman has changed a lot in the past and he's revealed his daily menu for body building on a couple of occasions. One version consists of cheese grits as well as poultry, egg white, and beef.

He's also displayed his diet during each of his work out video clip. In one video clip, he eats a lot of hamburger with loads of barbecue sauce on everything and drinks a Sprite/ grapes juice mix that happen to be not really the most typical meals when you think about eating clean.

A few of the rules include 2 grams of protein per lb of body weight (600 grams per day and 100 grams per meal.) He eats 6 meals per day and his major types of proteins are chicken, steak and turkey.

JAY CUTLER

His calorie goal is almost 4,700 per day, tries to keep his macros around 40/40/20.Cutler also consumes lots of poultry and brown rice, and states that about 5-6 hours of his day are spent cooking and eating. That is an outrageous time per day and is much more complicated to do constantly than any exercise.

Jay even awakens in the night to eat more because he states he often drops approximately 10 pound while he is sleeping. Almost all of his carbohydrates come from simple carbs due to the fact he says his size reduces with complex carbs.

Some of his older nutrition plans included plenty of oats and sweet potatoes but his current plans appears to have replaced them with white and brown rice. He consumes approximately 2 pounds of chicken and beef daily and prefers 2 glasses of egg white each morning with Ezekiel toast.

DORIAN YATES

Yates suggests 1- 1.5 grams of protein per pound of body weight and suggests double that for the carbohydrates.
His fat recommendation is around a third of the protein intake. Someone consuming 300 grams of proteins would get 600 grams of carbs and 100 grams of fat for a total of 4500 calories.

CHOOSING THE RIGHT DIET

Before you can come up with a diet plan to get started with, you have to know where you're at. It's essential to discover a specific technique to keep track of your weight and body fat percentage. Weight alone won't tell you how you're doing and neither will the body fat percentage, but when these 2 are mixed it can give you a fairly exact way to monitor your fat mass and body mass.

If you're not able to keep track of how you're progressing it is going to be hard to make changes in your specific eating plan because it will be challenging to know if the weight you gain is from muscle or fat.

SAMPLE MEAL PLAN- 2,500 CALORIES

The following is a sample 2,500-calorie diet plan. A 2,500-calorie diet plan is good for someone with a weight of 180 - 200 lbs. If you weight less than 180, eat somewhat less calories. If you weight more than 200 lbs, eat somewhat more calories. This plan represents that you sustain an active lifestyle.

Breakfast	**3 eggs omelet with spinach+ 1 cup oatmeal (550 calories)**
Lunch	Wild salmon+ potatoes + broccoli (550 calories)
Snack	50 grams whey protein (250 calories)
Post Workout Meal	Chicken + lentils+ brown rice (750 calories)
Dinner	Walnuts + cottage cheese (400 calories)

CHAPTER 4

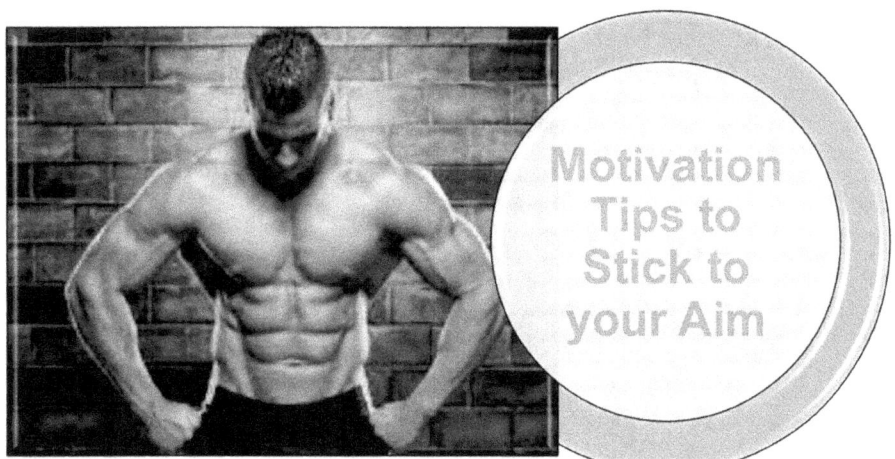

If you are interested in training your muscles harder and getting them in shape, then you have to encourage yourself for deep struggle and to stay on the right track, because several things can distract you from your goal.

Here are some tips that can help you to stick to your aim:

SELF-MOTIVATION

Self-motivation is a technique to encourage yourself to stick with your training and totally focus on your goal instead of being ripped in days. Inspire yourself from the legends of bodybuilding and never think, "I cannot achieve that body", rather you need to think, "Why I can't get a body shape like them?"

Never waste your time in observing other people; you should focus on your aim and workouts instead.

Listening to your favorite music and watching inspiring movies can motivate you to stay on the right track and to struggle hard to achieve your goal.Listening to your favorite music and watching inspiring movies can motivate you to stay on the right track and to struggle hard to achieve your goal.

AVOID OVERDO

Avoid overdo while exercising with your weights to build bigger and stronger muscles. Practicing or exercising more than your ability can degrade your muscles instead of developing. Exercising more than your ability often leads to fatigue that makes us less confident and reduces physical alertness throughout the day. Practicing high intensity exercises like working out with weights in the gym on consecutive days of the week can destruct your muscles instead of developing them.

Avoid overdo by practicing with heavy weights not more than three days a week to recover and build newer muscles naturally.

POWER YOUR BODY BY REDUCING EXTRA FAT

Keep yourself fit and de-stress by reducing unnecessary body fat. Unnecessary body fat leads to low energy while lifting weights to build bigger and stronger muscles and slows down muscle building process as well. Each one of aware of the dangers of unnecessary body fat, because unnecessary body fat is linked with several chronic health conditions. Burn unnecessary body fat through aerobic exercises in the days when you skip weight training. This is the main technique used by the most popular professionals. Simply, build muscles to burn body fat or burn your body fat to build stronger muscles.

FOCUS ON PROGRESSION

Try not to focus on perfection just focus on your progression to stay motivated. Focusing on perfection never allows you to change the ideas about bodybuilding techniques and old mindsets. Making a little good changes for exerting more stress on your muscles helps you developing bigger and stronger muscles faster than before. Getting your expected results in expected time is the successful conclusion of your goal. Focusing only on perfection will slow you down and keep you on a lazy and old traditional track that will soon distract you from the right track.

DAILY RITUALS

Make some of the most important exercises as you daily rituals to keep your body young, energetic and flexible that is the spirit of exercises. Here are some exercises that should be included in your daily rituals:

- Stretching or flexibility exercises
- A proper warm-up before your workouts and warm-down after your workout to attain an athletic performance
- Practice core exercises routinely, as these exercises improve overall strength and core stability that leads to a great muscle balance and endurance
- Meditate for better concentration on your workouts and to improve your inner abilities

MAKE AN ALGORITHM OF YOUR BIG GOAL

In the algorithm, a computer programmer divides a big problem into different smaller problems and solve them sequentially. Similarly, you just have to divide your big goal into different smaller ones and sequentially achieve them through your struggle. Setting big goals let you feel sorry for what you do not accomplish. Setting easier and smaller goals gives you true happiness and makes you realize that you can achieve a big goal too. For example, setting a goal like "I want to gain 20 pounds in only 5 days" will disappoint you and it will lessen your self-confidence and trust.

HAVE A LOOK ON YOUR MISTAKES

Do not ignore your mistakes, because "*one, who never feels remorse for his mistakes, remains unreformed for life*" or "*reformation is for one who admits his/her mistakes*". Let others (who are experienced and have achieved their goals) to correct your mistakes and try to learn from everyone, but focus on your decided goals is the key to stay on your goal and success.

ENTERTAIN YOURSELF

Entertain yourself by taking a recovery period of at least one week or less every two/three months to relax your brain from hard and struggling routine. Spend your recovery period by doing nothing just enjoying a healthy diet and healthy visiting (no exercises at all just relax). You can practice meditative exercises to boost up your concentration and to awaken pre-awareness.

TRAINING PARTNER

A partner for your training is the one who can help you in achieving your goals. Get a training partner, because a partner is the best motivation for you. Your partner can encourage you when he feels that the task is bigger than your abilities.

ALTERNATE COMBINATIONS

Your bodybuilding career is going on the wheels of your exercise routine. So, keep changing these tires to run this career safely. I mean change your exercise routine by making a little bit change in your routine combination. Performing flat bench and incline bench press one combination and incline bench press and parallel bar dips another combination is a good change you can make in your exercise plan.

ALWAYS THINK ABOUT THE BIG REWARD

Make a routine exercises plan with an effective combination and always keep in mind your big reward you always want to achieve through bodybuilding and then start your workouts. Thinking about the big reward before starting the everyday workout, instill the true spirit of athletic performance and enthusiasm.

CHAPTER 5

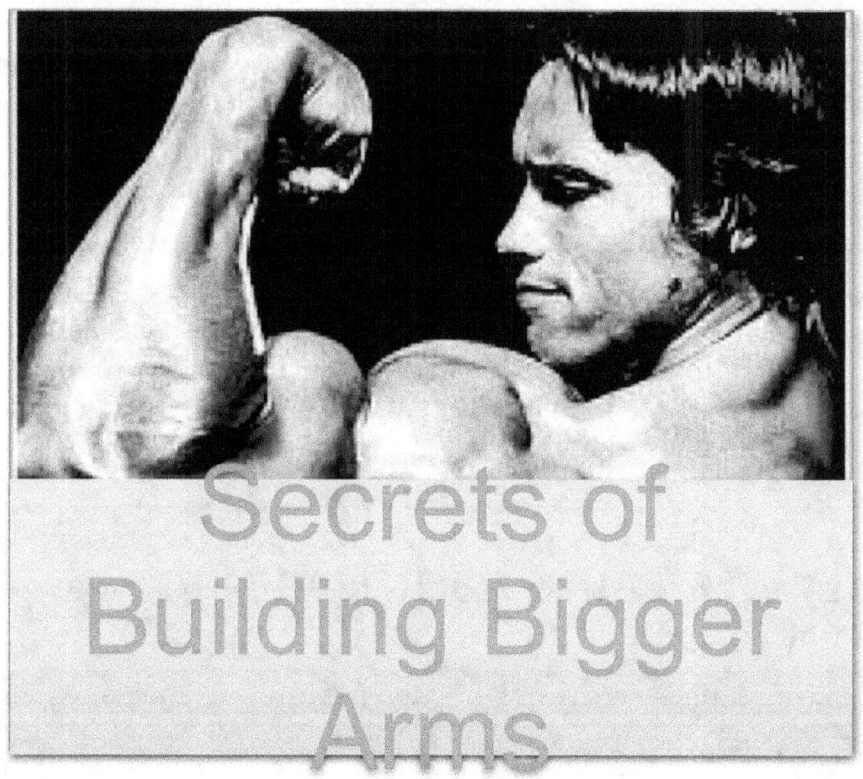

As described earlier that bigger muscles can be achieved through multiple steps, therefore we have to follow all these steps build bigger and well-defined arms. The secrets of developing bigger arms have now revealed. In this chapter, we will discuss an appropriate way of developing muscular arms.

STEP BY STEP PROGRESS

The bodybuilding legends adopted different techniques to build bigger and stronger arms as they all have different body mechanics. Therefore, you should learn some movement patterns and get past beginner stages to completely understand your body mechanics and then move to the next goal. If you have built stamina, power and muscle coordination, then it is the right time to become a monster, but you still have to struggle for it. To learn various techniques of developing amazing and bigger muscles especially bigger arms, you have to spend hours in the gym. To achieve an athletic performance and to build Hulk's arms it is necessary to develop base level of strength.

HIT THE IRON WHEN IT IS HOT

Do not make haste in achieving your goal, because bigger dreams never come true quickly. Progression requires time and struggle, so you need to stick to your plan and working hard on workout techniques mentioned in previous chapters. Do heavy weight exercises first and low weight exercises later to focus on your arm muscles properly. The best mass-building exercises should be performed early in the workout to avoid low energy level and to perform your workout with ease and enthusiasm.

In the beginning, a workout seems like it really works, but after a while when your body becomes habitual to this workout, then the strength and growth of your arms or other muscles starts to slow down. It is the right time to change intensity and weights in your routine workouts. Doing the same workouts will stop the growth and strength of your muscles.

Here are some tips to develop bigger arms:

- Do a proper warm up as needed, but avoid take warm-up sets to muscle failure

- Choose a weight to reach muscle failure by the target reps

- Try to complete a set between 30 to 50 seconds, as the sweet spot seems to be between 30 to 50 seconds per set

- Do your one rep in 4 to 5 seconds to make your training much tougher and effective

- Void any sort of exercise on recovery days or off days (not even cardio exercises)

ARM EXERCISES

Here are some effective workouts based on Arnold inspired training you should perform;

Parallel bar triceps dips 6-8 reps, 3-4 sets
Barbell biceps curl 6-8 reps, 3-4 sets
Close grip bench press 6-8 reps, 3-4 sets
Dumbbell biceps curl 6-8 reps, 3-4 sets
Cable triceps pushdown 6-8 reps, 3-4 sets
Cable biceps curl 6-8 reps, 3-4 sets
Ball throwing (optional) 15-20 reps, 3-4 set

FINISH

Thank you again for downloading this book!

I hope this book was able to help you improve your health and physique.

The next step is to apply what you learned and take massive amount of action.

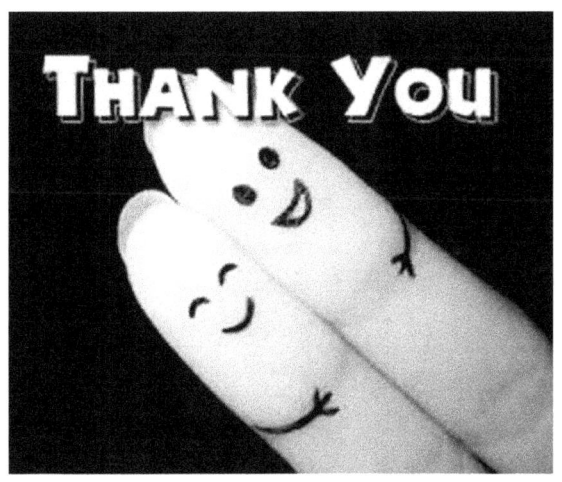

Finally, if you enjoyed this book, then I'd like to ask you for a favor, would you be kind enough to leave a review for this book on Amazon? It'd be greatly appreciated!

Thank you and good luck!

Check my other book on amazon.com
Amazon.com/author/arnoldyates